Some Secrets
Should Never Be Kept

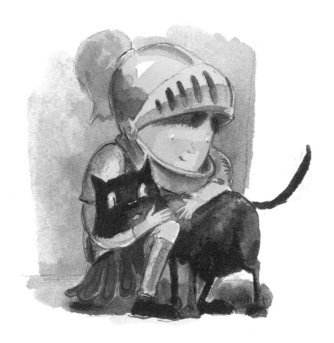

*Protect children from unsafe touch by
teaching them to always speak up*

by **Jayneen Sanders**

illustrated by **Craig Smith**

Note from the author

As the mother of three young children, I knew at some stage in their young lives I would not be there to protect them. With the talk of the 'first sleep-over', it became clear I needed to broach the delicate subject of how they could protect themselves from inappropriate touch. I challenged myself to write this book so parents, caregivers and educators had a tool (one I did not have) to open up the discussion on self-protection. Forewarned is forearmed. If a situation like the one Sir Alfred encountered were to happen to a child, it is my sincere hope that they could draw on what they have learned from the story and the subsequent, essential discussion — and speak up.

Jayneen Sanders is the mother of three daughters, a teacher and an author.

Some Secrets Should Never Be Kept
Educate2Empower Publishing an imprint of
UpLoad Publishing Pty Ltd
Victoria Australia
www.upload.com.au

First published in 2011
Reprinted in 2013
Reprinted in 2017

Text copyright © Jayneen Sanders 2011
Illustration copyright © Craig Smith 2011

Written by Jayneen Sanders
Cover illustration and illustrations by Craig Smith
Designed by Susannah Low, Butterflyrocket Design

Some Secrets Should Never Be Kept :
Protect children from unsafe touch by
teaching them to always speak up

ISBN: 9780987186010 (paperback)

Dedication

To my husband and children who encourage me in everything I do. JS

To the children who suffer —
be brave and tell. JS

For George Tetlow,
who turned me on to drawing. CS

Note to the reader

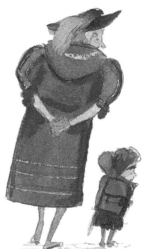

It is important that young children are educated in personal safety and to speak up if they are touched inappropriately. Here are some general 'Body Safety' tips, followed by more specific guidelines on reading *Some Secrets Should Never Be Kept* to your child.

General Body Safety Tips

- Young children often find it hard to articulate how they are feeling. Therefore, provide daily opportunities to talk about feelings. Ask questions such as, *How do you feel when it's your birthday? When you pat a puppy? When you go down a big slide for the first time?*

- Discuss 'safe' and 'unsafe' feelings and brainstorm scenarios. Discuss how your child feels when they are worried or unsafe. Talk about what happens to their body: sweaty hands, racing heart, start to cry, sick in their tummy, wobbly knees, etc. Say, *These are your Early Warning Signs and they tell you when something is not right.* Encourage your child to always tell a trusted adult if they experience their Early Warning Signs.

- Introduce the term 'private body parts'. Tell your child that their private body parts are the areas under their bathing suit. Use the correct terminology for body parts from a young age. Tell your child that no-one can touch their private body parts (which also includes their mouth) and they can say 'Stop!' or 'No!' if someone does. Reinforce that they should tell someone they trust about the inappropriate touch. Have your child practise putting out their hand and saying 'Stop!' or 'No!' Tell your child that it is also wrong for them to touch somebody else's private parts, even if they are asked to, and if they see pictures of private parts they should tell a trusted adult. Discuss when it is appropriate for someone to touch their body, e.g. a doctor, but only if you or a trusted adult is in the room.

Reading 'Some Secrets Should Never Be Kept'

1 Explain to your child that you are going to read a very special story. Show the cover and read the title. Ask, *Who do you think this little boy is? How do you think he is feeling? Why do you think he is feeling this way?*

2 Read the story, stopping and discussing the illustrations when appropriate. *Note*: in the first reading, we suggest that you keep the discussion of the illustrations brief, so that the storyline is not lost. Once the story is finished, go straight to the Discussion Questions at the back of the book. Spend as long as appropriate on each question. *Note*: when reading the story again, discuss the little boy's body language and ask your child how the little boy might be feeling.

3 Revisit the story in the following week. Say, *Do you remember this story? What was it about? What happened to the boy? Should we keep secrets such as someone touching our private parts? What Early Warning Signs did the little boy have? What would you do if someone touched your private parts?* Reinforce to your child that they have the right to tell the person to stop, and that it is important to tell someone they trust and keep on telling until they are believed.

4 Continuing on from this discussion, have your child name three to five adults that they could tell if they are feeling unsafe or experiencing their Early Warning Signs. Talk about how these people are part of their 'Safety Network' — people who they trust and who will always believe them.

5 Revisit the story every few months or when a situation arises where your child is in the care of another person. Reinforce the key messages: your body is *your* body and no-one has the right to touch it, and secrets that make you feel bad and uncomfortable should never be kept.

For more children's books and information on this topic go to: www.e2epublishing.info

Remember: Forewarned is forearmed! Please encourage others to teach Body Safety.

In a land not so far away, lived
a brave little knight.

Sir Alfred, for that was his name, lived in a teeny
weeny cottage with his mother, Lady Susan.

Lady Susan had once lived a fabulous and
glamorous life, but since her divorce from
Sir Alfred's father they were now quite poor.

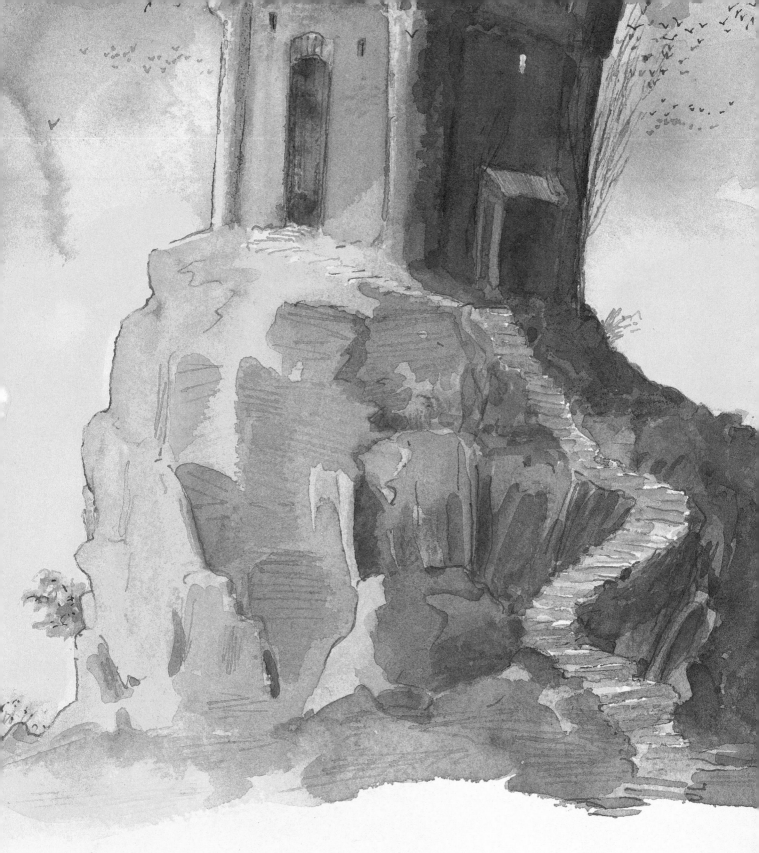

Lady Susan worked very hard day after day, cleaning
the largest castle in the land. The castle was owned
by the rich and famous Lord Henry Votnar.

Because Alfred was only a little knight and couldn't stay home alone, he always went to Lord Henry's castle after school. While Lady Susan continued to clean and scrub, Lord Henry offered to take care of Alfred.

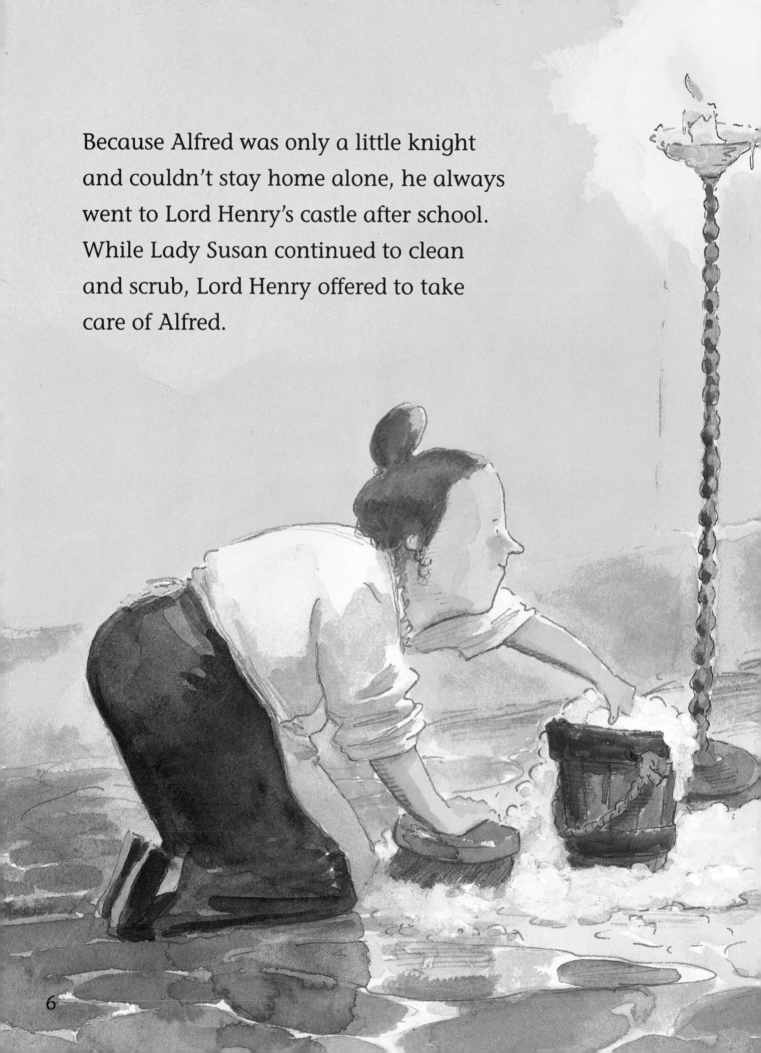

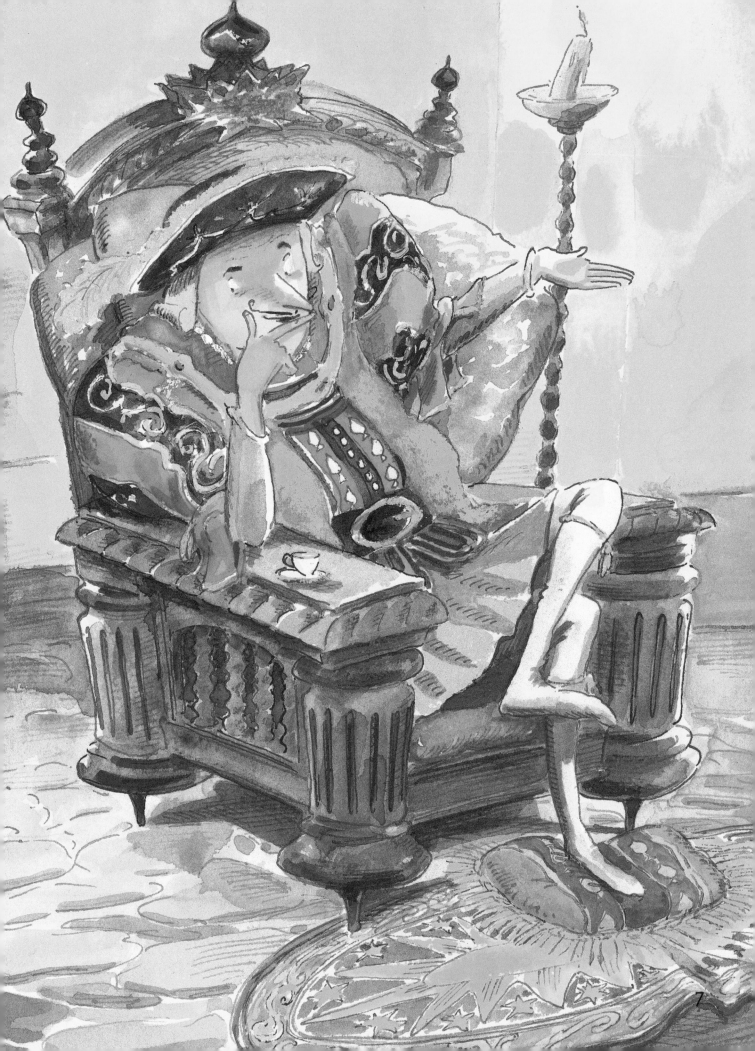

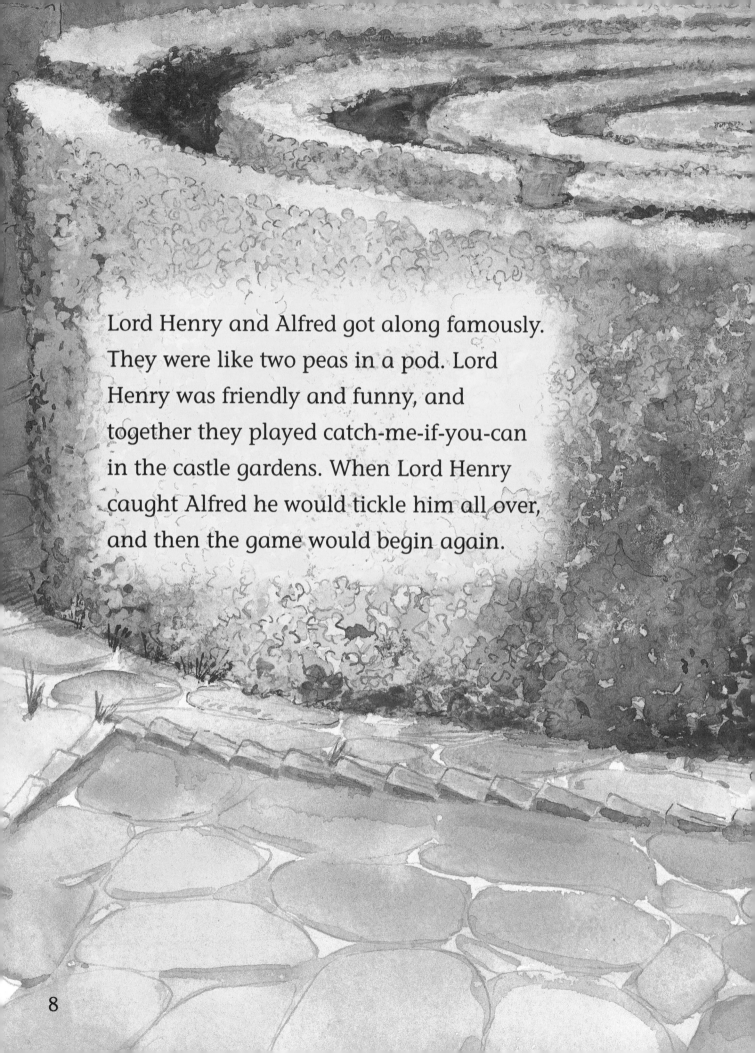

Lord Henry and Alfred got along famously. They were like two peas in a pod. Lord Henry was friendly and funny, and together they played catch-me-if-you-can in the castle gardens. When Lord Henry caught Alfred he would tickle him all over, and then the game would begin again.

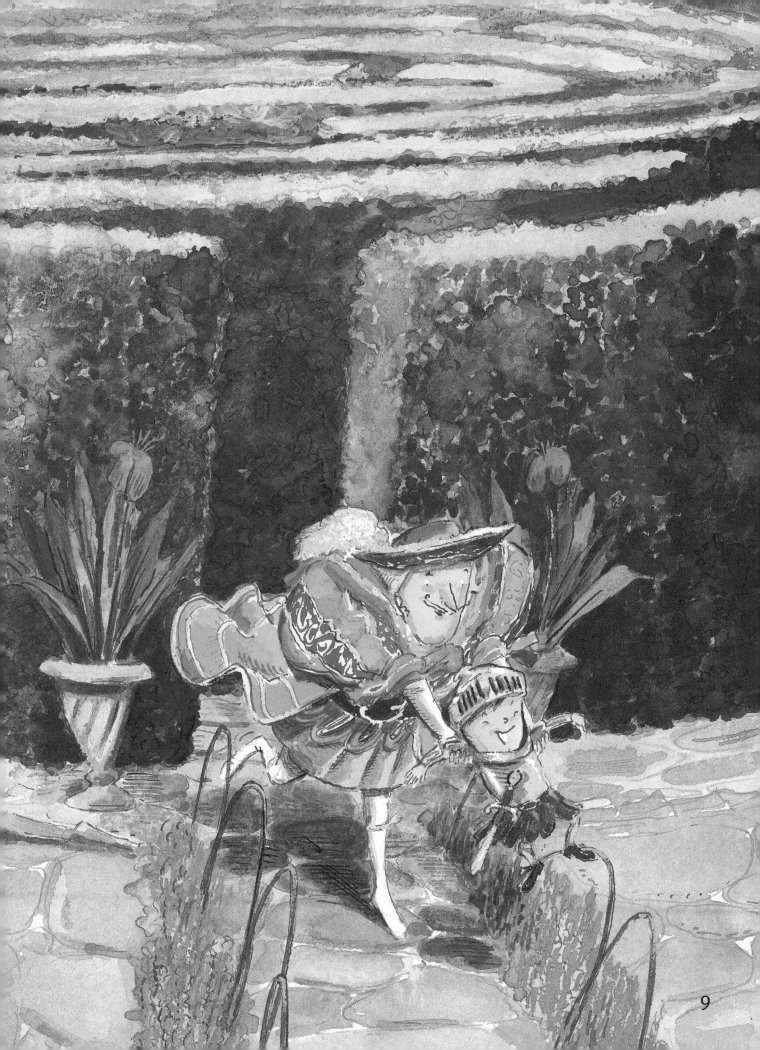

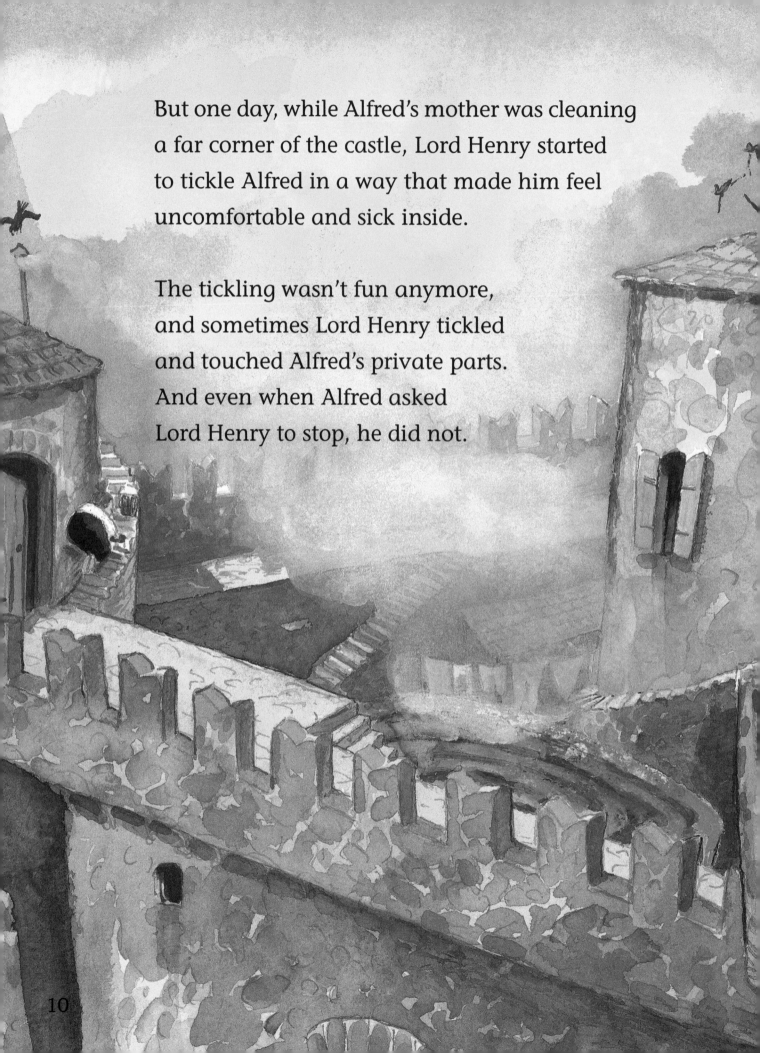

But one day, while Alfred's mother was cleaning
a far corner of the castle, Lord Henry started
to tickle Alfred in a way that made him feel
uncomfortable and sick inside.

The tickling wasn't fun anymore,
and sometimes Lord Henry tickled
and touched Alfred's private parts.
And even when Alfred asked
Lord Henry to stop, he did not.

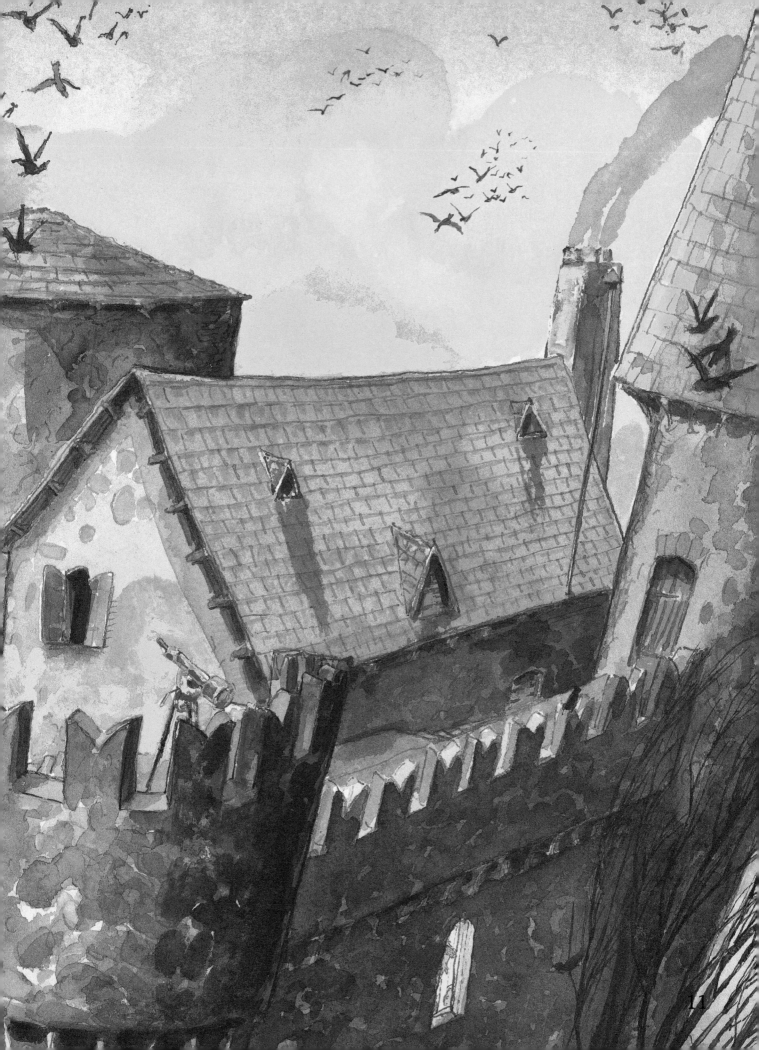

11

"Come on, Alfred," laughed Lord Henry. "It's just a bit of fun. There's no harm in a bit of tickling."

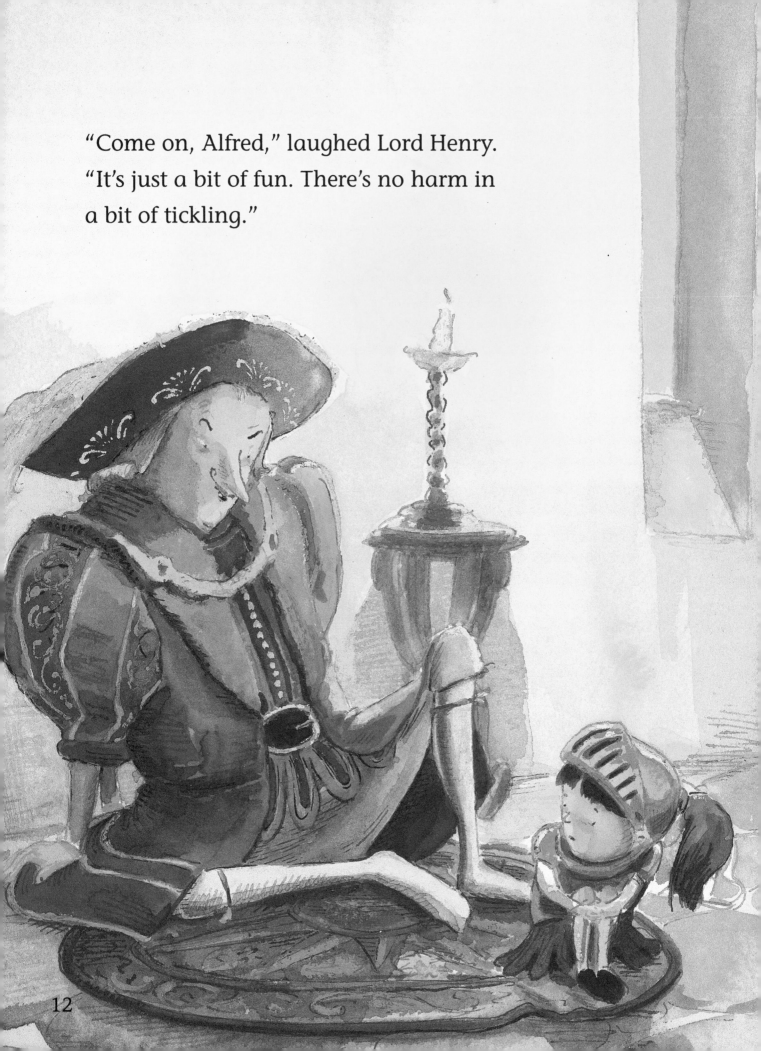

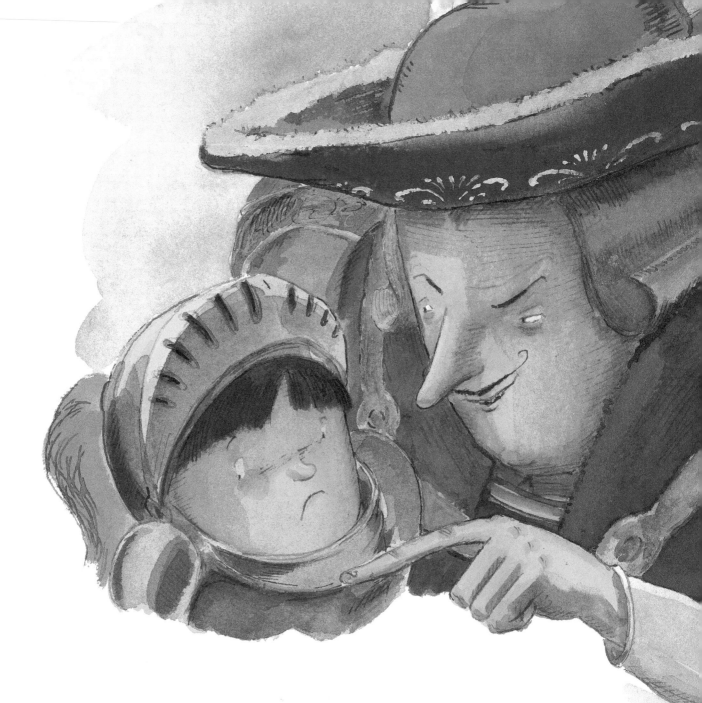

"But," warned Lord Henry, "you must never ever tell anyone about our tickling game. It must be our special secret. Because..." continued Lord Henry, "if you do tell, I'm afraid your mother will not be able to clean my castle anymore, and you will have no money for food and clothes and... it will be all YOUR fault, Alfred."

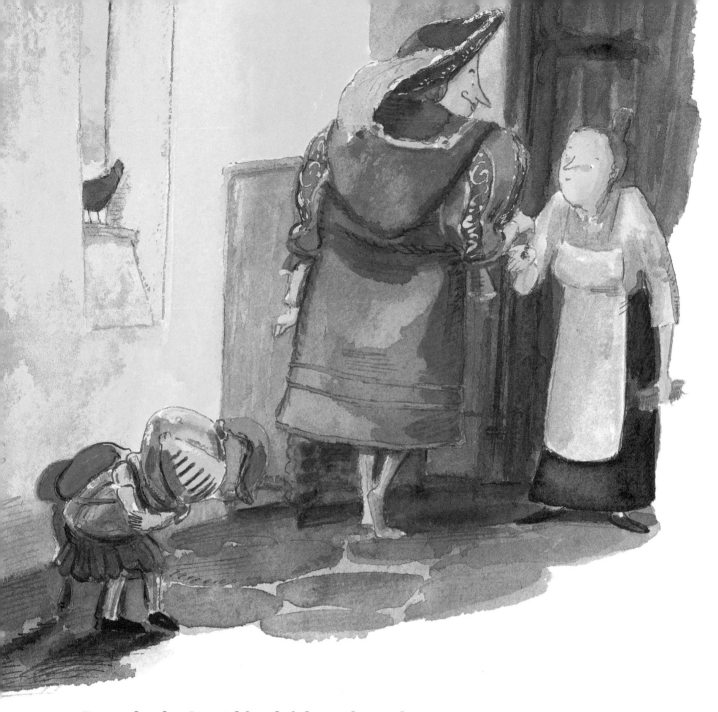

Poor little Sir Alfred felt sick with worry.
He knew some secrets should NEVER EVER
be kept — secrets that made him feel bad and
uncomfortable. Secrets just like this. But if he
told anyone, his mother would lose her job
and they would have no money. And the worst
bit of all — it would be all his fault.

That night, little Sir Alfred went home with a very heavy heart. He did not eat his supper and he barely spoke a word to his mother. He crawled into his bed feeling sad and lonely — the secret heavy in his heart.

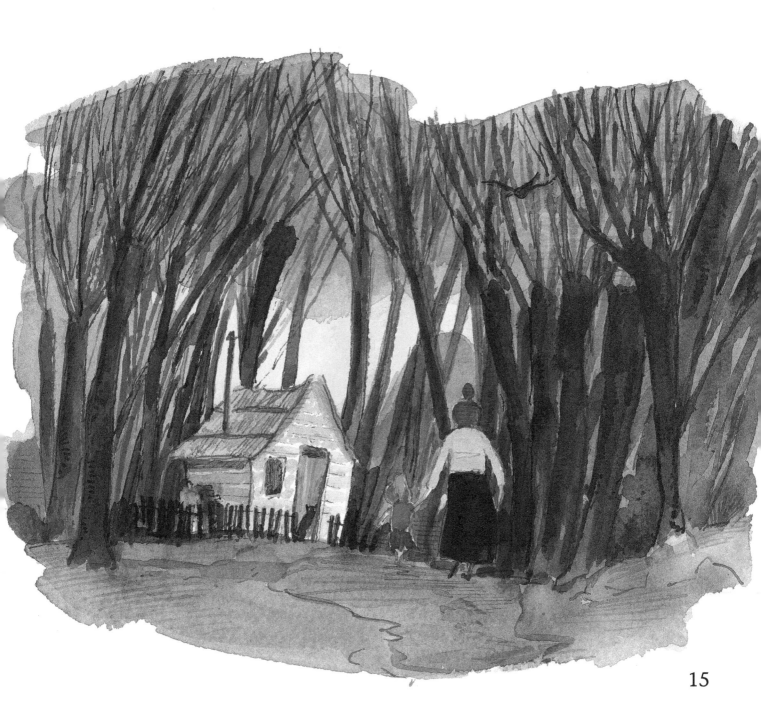

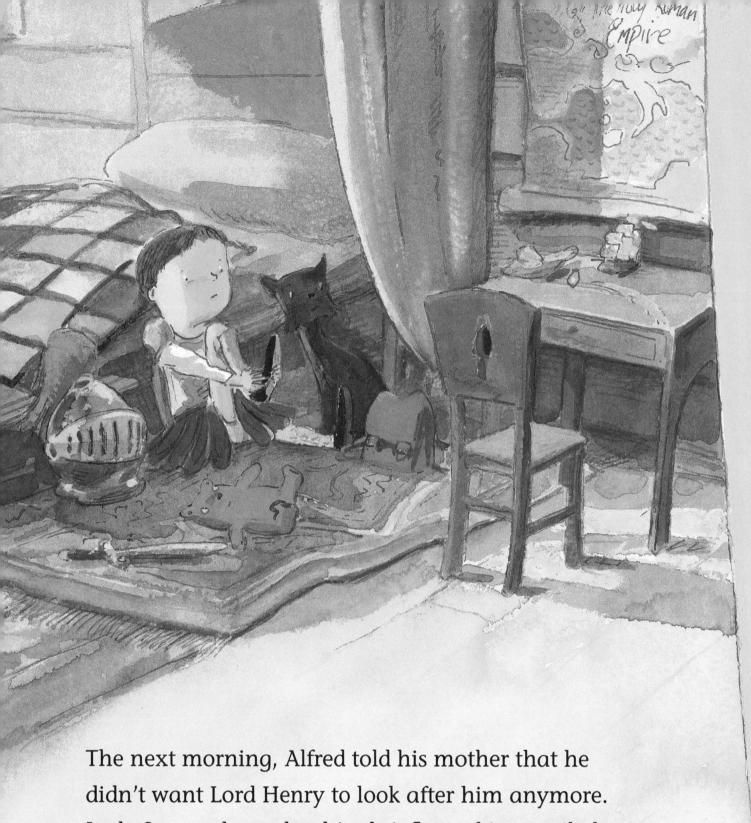

The next morning, Alfred told his mother that he didn't want Lord Henry to look after him anymore. Lady Susan glanced at him briefly and just smiled, "Don't be a silly billy, Alfred. Everyone loves Lord Henry. He is one of the nicest and kindest men in the world. We are very lucky he takes care of you."

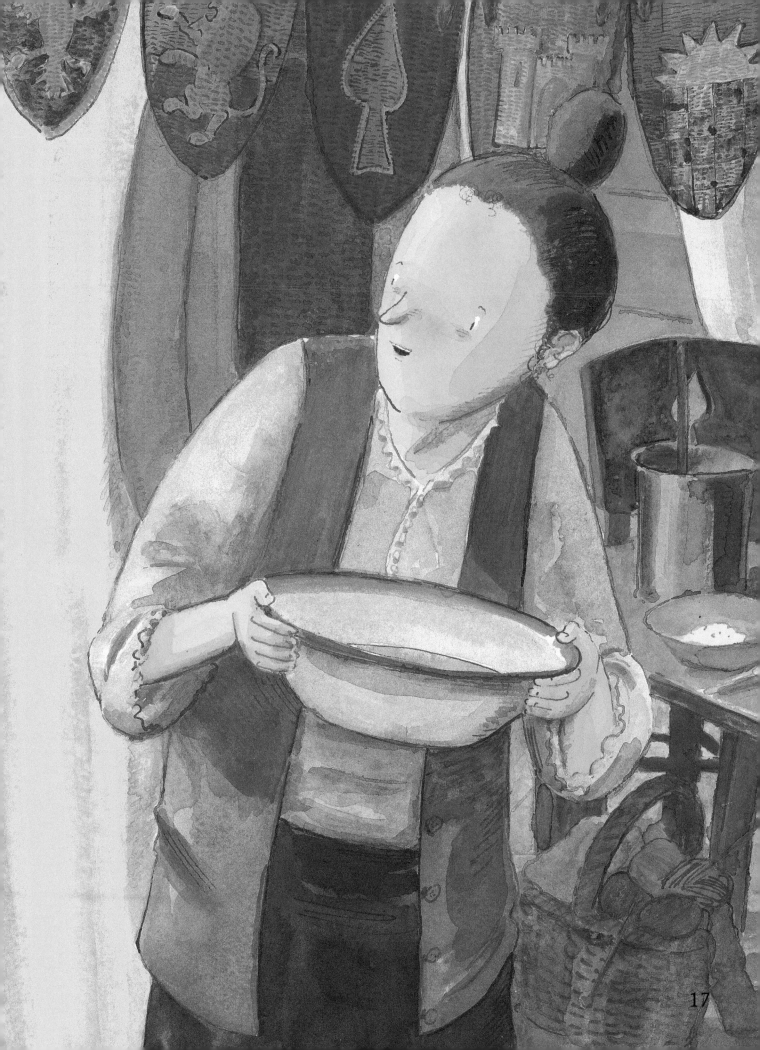

17

But that afternoon when Lord Henry came to the school gate, Alfred felt sick in his tummy. He felt scared and very confused. He didn't want his mother to lose her job, so once again Lord Henry tickled him and touched his private parts.

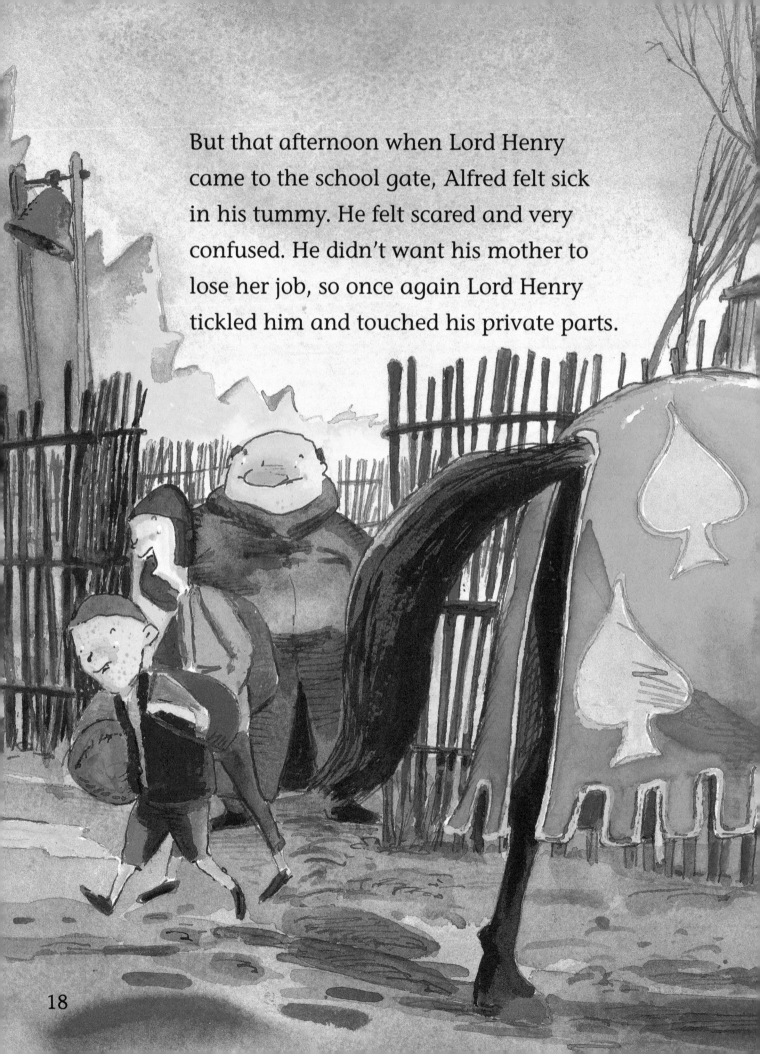

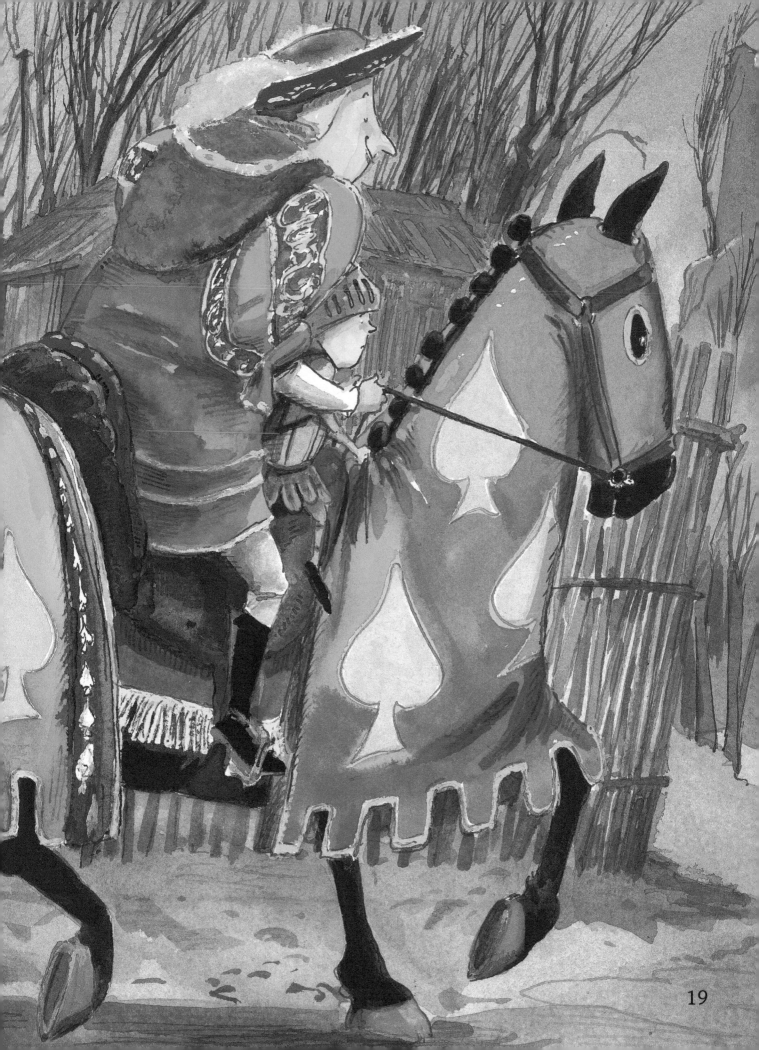

When Alfred arrived home that evening,
he felt so ill that he went straight to bed.
As he lay in the dark of his room, he cried
and cried. Great sobs lifted up and out of his
heart. He felt so lonely and so frightened.

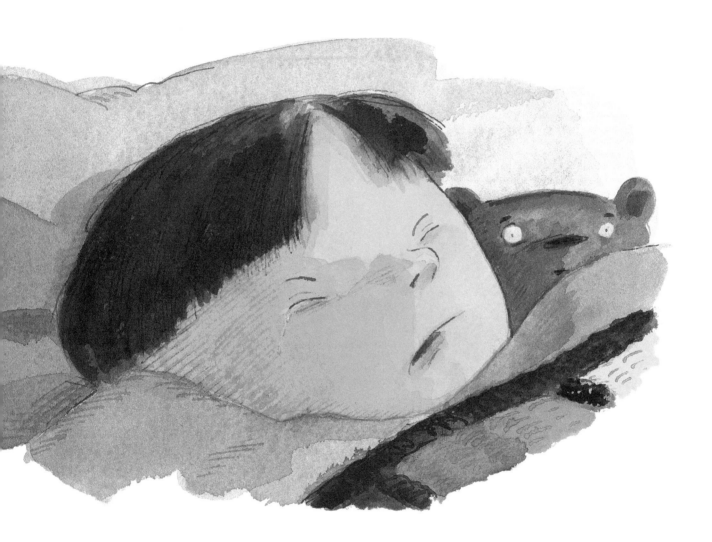

From her rocking chair in the kitchen, Lady Susan
could hear Alfred sobbing. She stopped her knitting
and went straight to her little son.

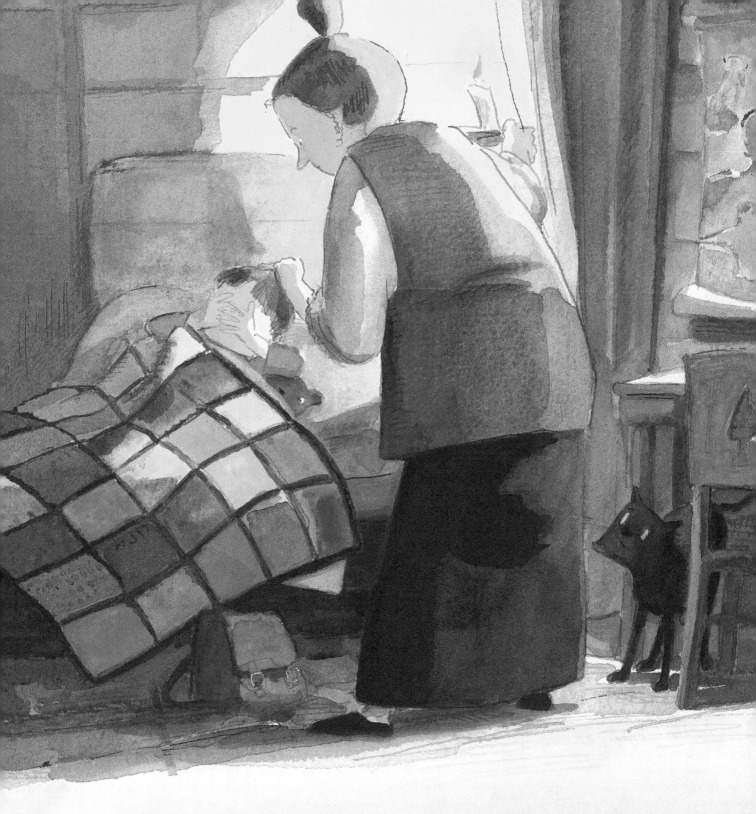

"Whatever is the matter?" she asked. But Alfred
did not utter a word. If he told his mother his
terrible secret, she would lose her job and they
would have no money and no food.

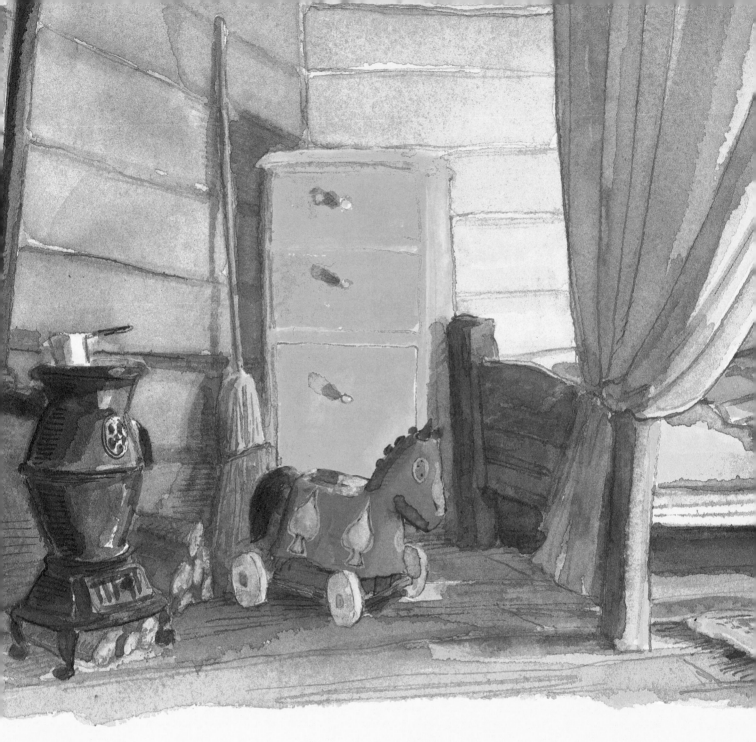

Lady Susan hugged her little boy in a loving
and gentle way. She held his face in her hands
and looked deep into his eyes. "There is nothing
you cannot tell me," she said. "Nothing at all.
I have always told you, Alfred, some secrets
should NEVER EVER be kept."

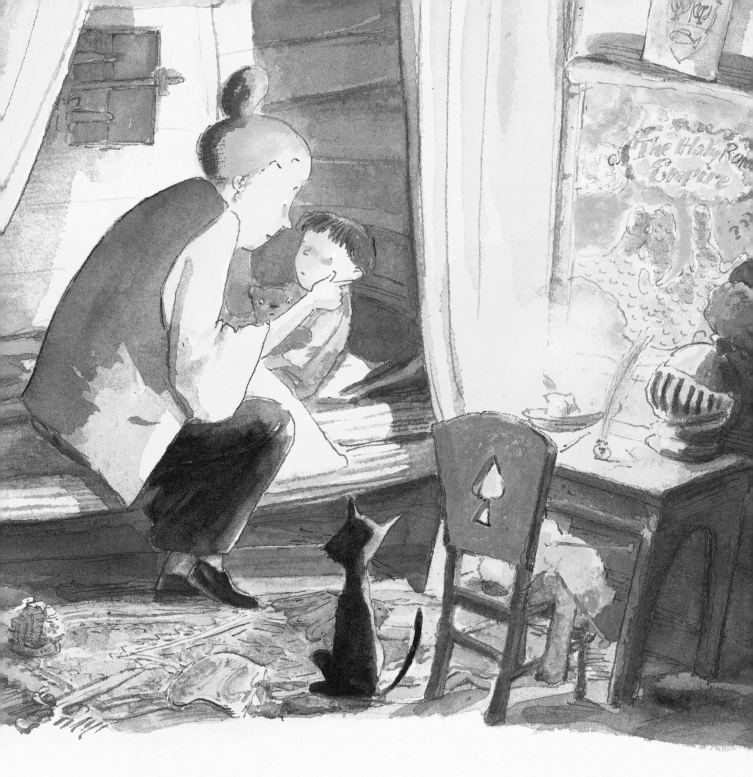

Poor little Sir Alfred was so confused. He didn't
know whether to tell his mother or not. What if
she didn't believe him? What if she lost her job
and he was to blame?

Finally, after many tears and lots of warm hugs from his mother, little Sir Alfred decided to be brave. He decided to tell the terrible secret.

Once he began, his words tumbled out one on top of the other. He told his mother all about the tickling and the touching, and how uncomfortable and sick it made him feel.

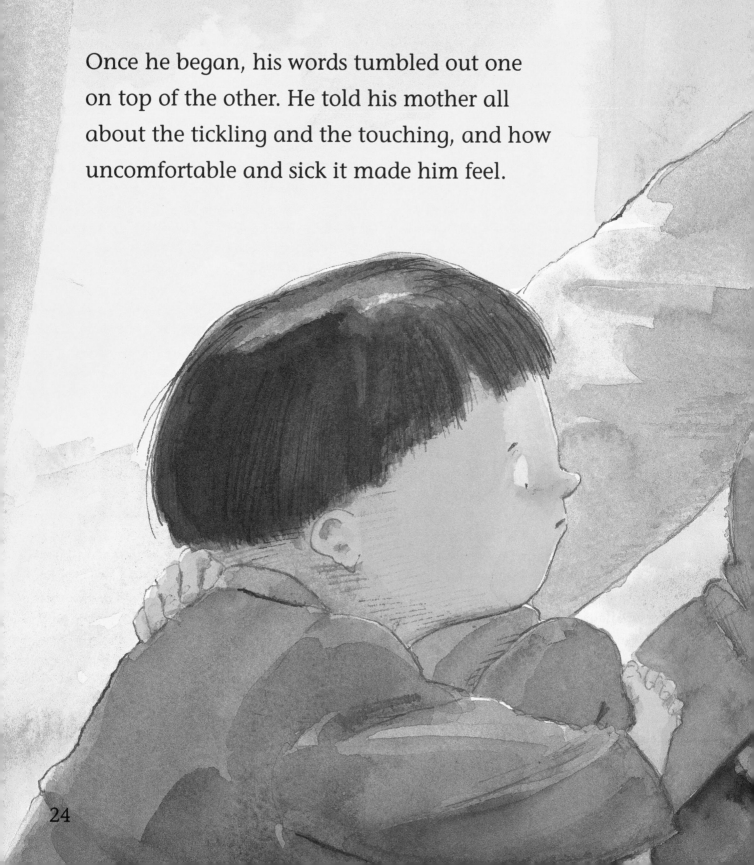

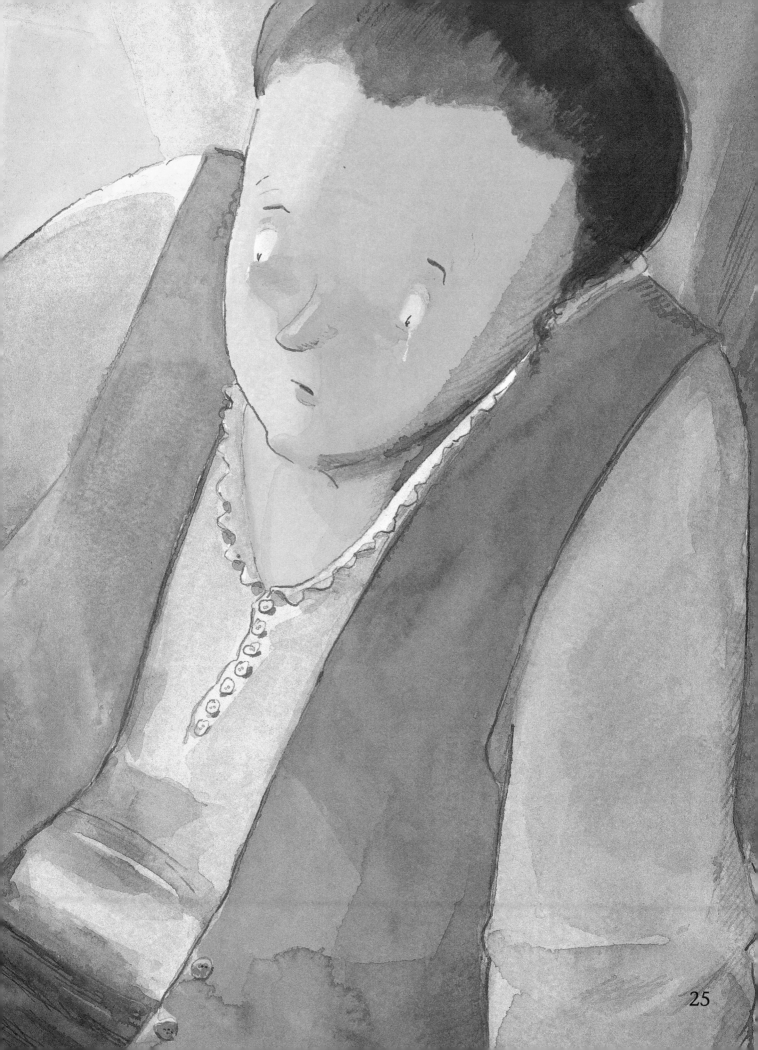

He told her that Lord Henry said he must keep
the secret, and that if he told anyone, Lady Susan
would lose her job and they would have no
money — and it would be all HIS fault.

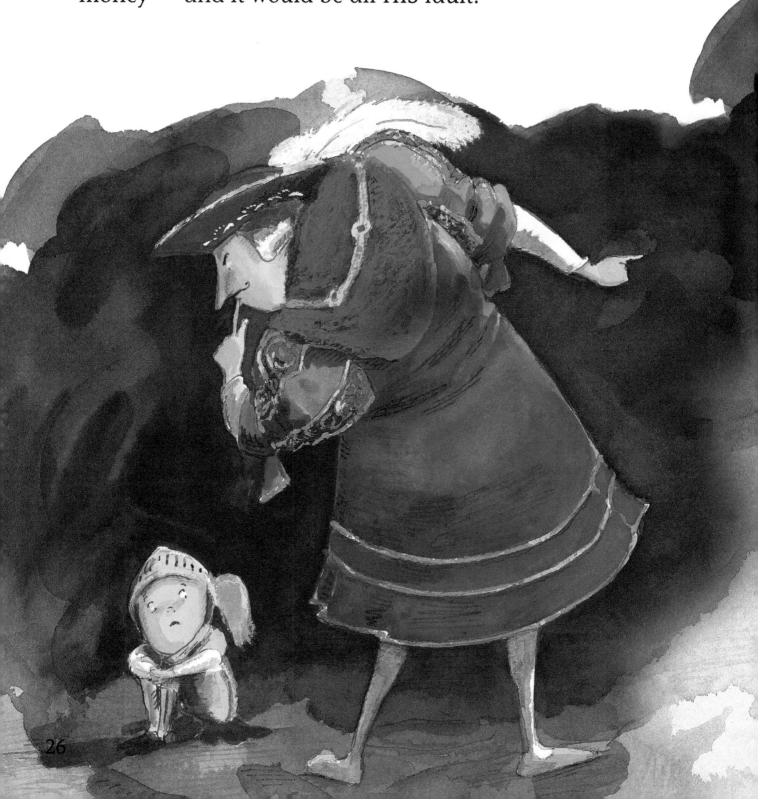

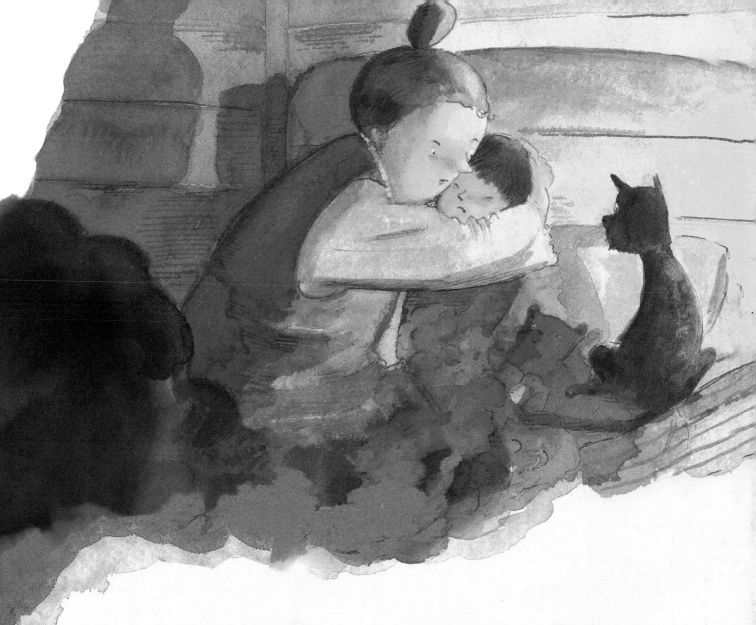

Lady Susan hugged her son very tightly and rocked him gently back and forth. At last she wiped away both their tears. "You are the bravest little knight I have ever known," she said, "and what Lord Henry did to you was very wrong. You were right to tell me and I am very proud of you — remember there is NOTHING you cannot tell me. I am always here to listen to you and I will ALWAYS believe you. YOU have done nothing wrong."

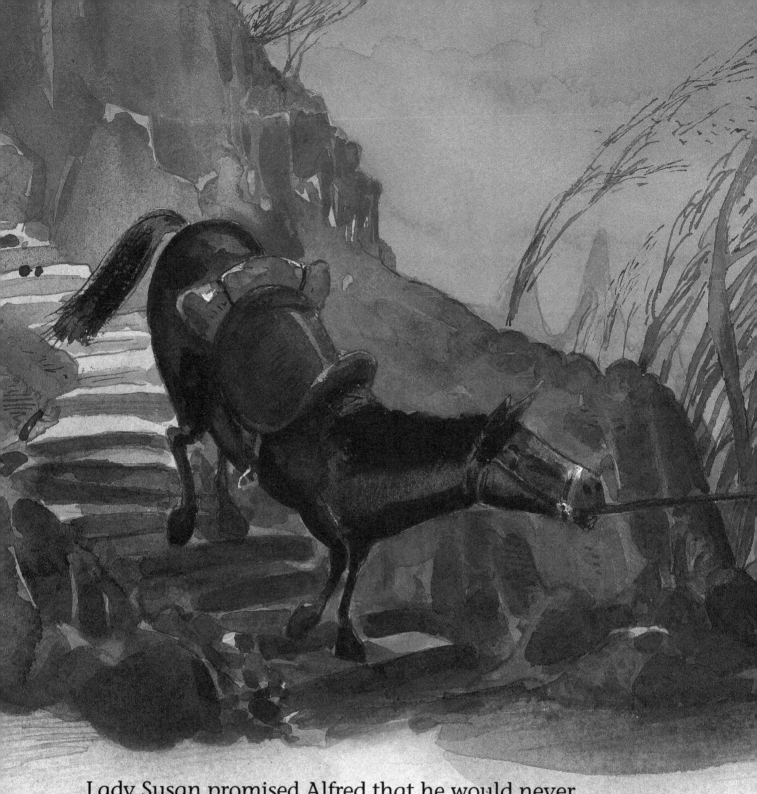

Lady Susan promised Alfred that he would never
ever have to see Lord Henry again, and that he would
be gone from their lives forever. As punishment,
Lord Henry would be banished from his castle and
the kingdom.

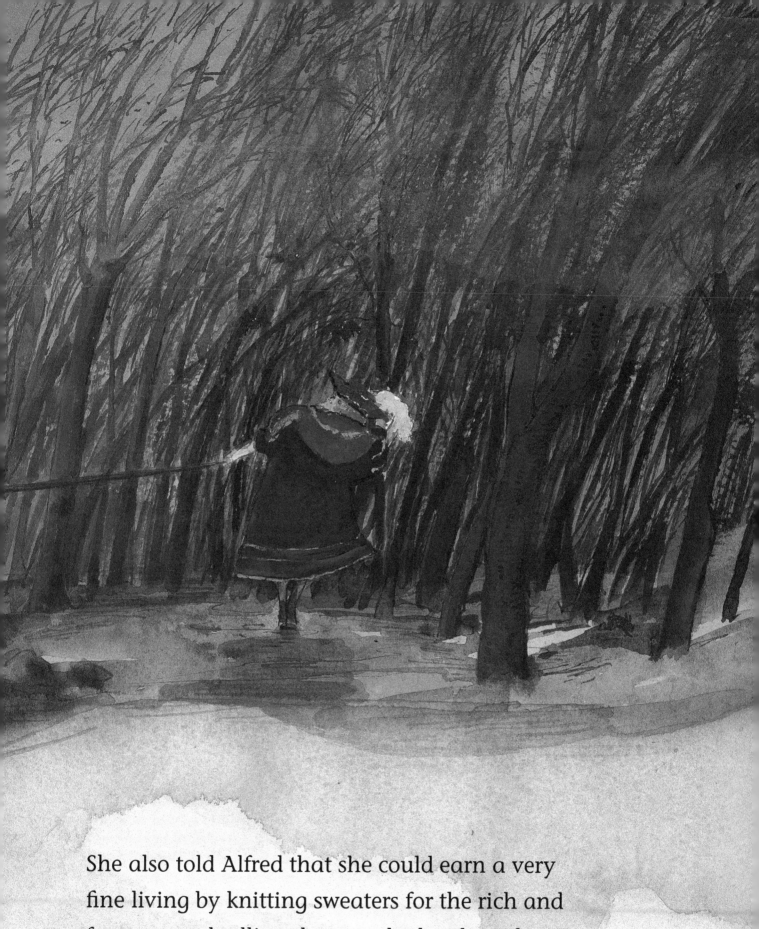

She also told Alfred that she could earn a very
fine living by knitting sweaters for the rich and
famous, and selling them at the local market.

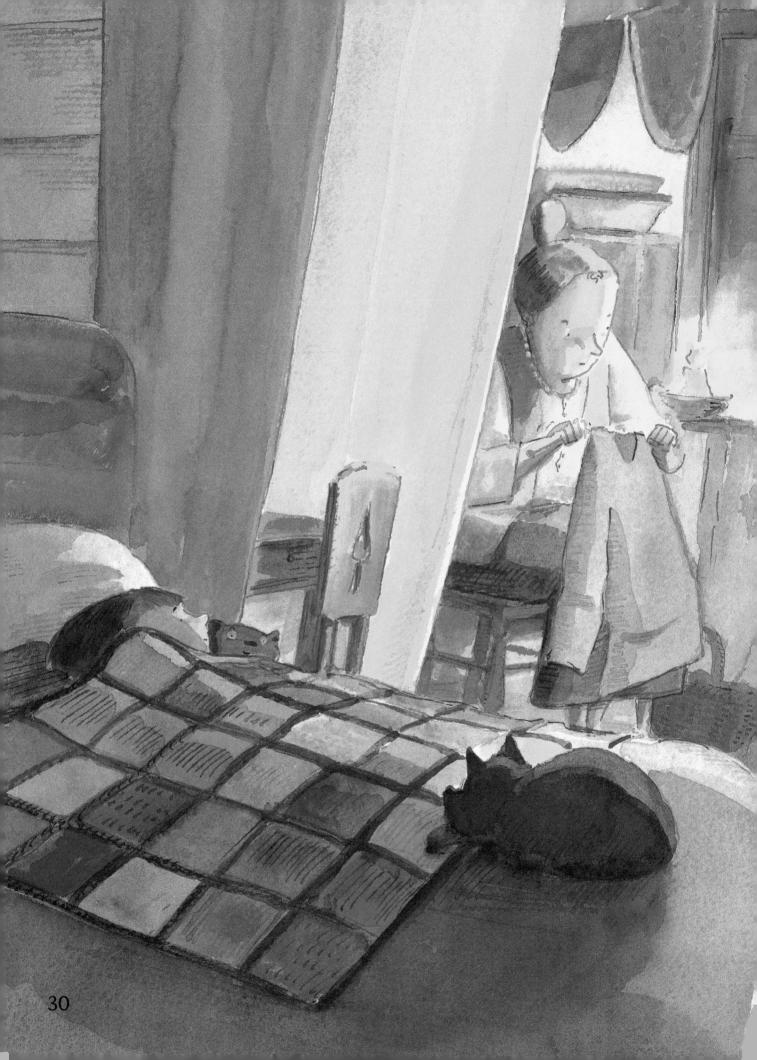

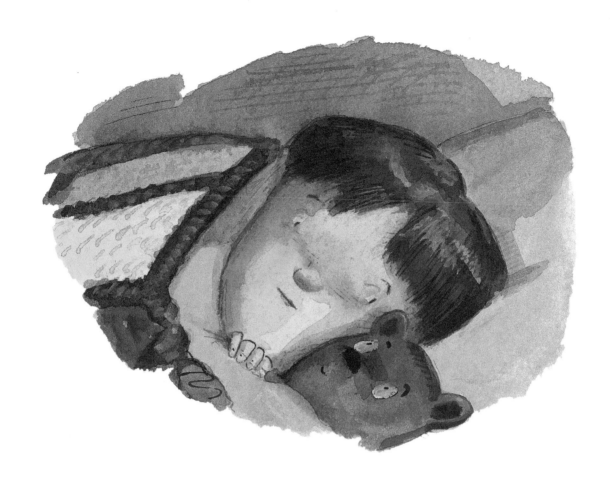

Later that night, as little Sir Alfred lay snug and warm in his bed, he finally felt safe and very loved. He was proud of himself because he had found the courage to tell his mother. He knew now, for sure, that no matter how awful or scary the secret, it should NEVER EVER be kept.

Discussion Questions
for Parents, Caregivers and Educators

When Lord Henry started to tickle Alfred in a way that he did not like, was Alfred right to tell him to stop? When Lord Henry did not stop, what should Alfred have done?

Why didn't Alfred tell his mother about the touching and tickling straightaway? How might Alfred have been feeling?

Should Alfred have told his mother straightaway?

Should anyone tickle or touch your private parts?

If they do, what should you do straightaway?

What if the person says it is "our special secret" — should you keep that kind of secret?

Sometimes there are good secrets (happy surprises), such as not telling your mother about a surprise birthday party, or not telling your grandpa about a present you have bought him. But sometimes there are unsafe secrets, such as someone touching your private parts. A secret such as this should never ever be kept. If someone tells you to keep an unsafe secret, what should you do?

Who could you tell? . . . Yes, that's right. You could tell someone you really trust, such as your mother or father, or your teacher, or even a much older brother or sister. Remember — some secrets should never ever be kept.

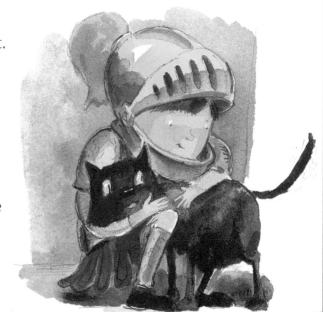

Have you got any questions about the story that you would like to ask?

For more information: www.e2epublishing.info

CPSIA information can be obtained
at www.ICGtesting.com
Printed in the USA
BVHW021454290622
640936BV00004B/91

9 780987 186010